SIX SECRETS FOR SURVIVING THE ICU

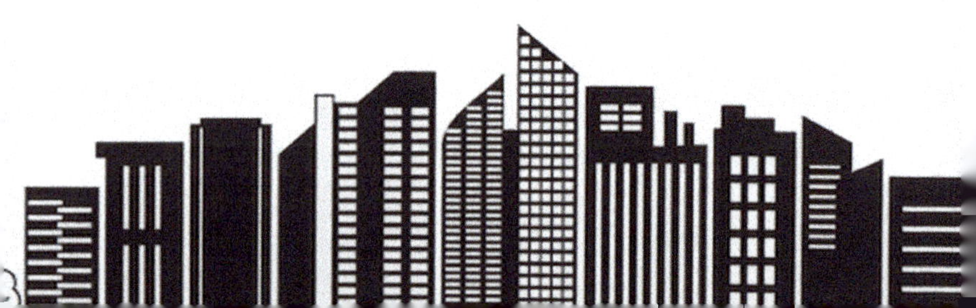

WIN
WOULD BE WON IF EVERYONE WON ONE, EVERYONE WOULD
1
www.win-one.org

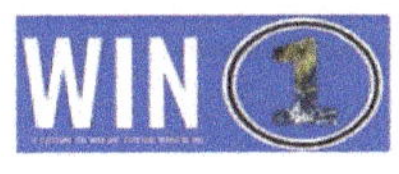
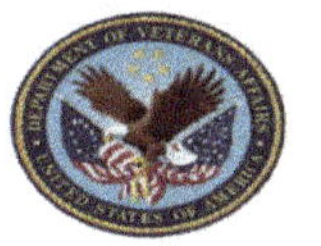
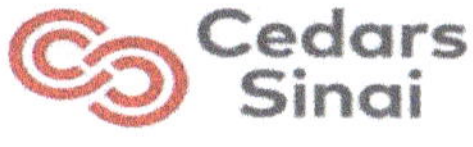

**From
"Thee Miracle Mann"
Designed by the Divine Team... Created at Cedars Sinai and the Veterans Affairs Hospital
Lewis D. Stallworth III**

Greetings my new friend!

It is a pleasure to meet you and hopefully help you. If you are reading this, it means that either you yourself, or a loved one that you care for, needs help. Furthermore, you also need to know how to get that help and what your options are? Especially if you find yourself in a situation needing an organ transplant or major surgery like I was in. If this sounds like you or the person you are advocating for, please keep reading as the following information can save lives.

The key to navigating a hospital is recognizing going in that hospital scares even the biggest and strongest of people. Let's start with my situation. I had four heart attacks, mainly due to high blood pressure. After diet, exercise, a passed psyche exam, and most importantly, having the proper team in place to support me, I was approved to receive both, a heart and kidney transplants on the same day, and ultimately given a new lease on life. Not bad, considering the first doctor I had assigned to me, basically issued me a death certificate. Fortunately for me, I wanted to live and I believed in myself more than that doctor ever did, and I stuck with it, figured out how to navigate the healthcare system, learned what options were available to me, found doctors with compassion at Cedars and the VA, who did believe in me, and now I'm here to empower you on how you can do it too.

Secret #1

The easiest way to learn about your status is by having someone on your team advocating for you, who knows how the healthcare system works.

The only way you're going to know your health status is if you have someone to trust, who's been through the system already. Just because you go into the hospital, doesn't mean you're necessarily going to be received by someone who is actually going to care for you. Hospitals are big businesses, if you don't have good health insurance, or are on Medi-Cal, it's their job to get you in and out, unless you know the right questions to ask. That is why the first step is having someone who knows the system and is ready to go in with you, drop you off at the hospital, pick you up, and take care of you afterwards.

I was fortunate to have a host of people advocating for me, but people also need to realize that even if you don't have family or friends to act as your caretaker, there are great social workers out there who will work with you every step of the way to ensure you have the proper healthcare team to tend to your needs. At every hospital, *right now there is a social worker waiting for you to call them, who wants to help you. They can co-ordinate everything for you from travel to and from the hospital, to in-home healthcare, but you also need to be patient, because at the end of the day, they're helping a lot more people than just you. If you trust the process though, those social workers will find you everything you need to succeed.*

Having someone advocating for you is critical to the process and that person having a good relationship with your primary care doctor can make all the difference in the world, especially if you are someone who is naturally quiet in public. Patients need to realize, every doctor and every social worker has so many people they're already working to help. If your answer to every question is, "I don't know," then nobody is going to want to help you. You must find a way to engage your doctors. That is why it is important that you have someone who you trust, who knows the system and can say for you what you might not be able to say.

Your caretakers need to be on the same page with your doctors too. Same goes for your doctors.

There's no guarantee that your doctors

are communicating with each other properly, and that is when your caretaker needs to step in and help ensure that everyone is on the same page when it comes to your treatment. It's important to realize that at different points you will need different people supporting you. Even if you are told "no" initially, find out why you were denied and then work with your team members and with the hospital social workers, because that "no" could become a "yes" later on down the road, if you stick to the program.

Secret #2:

If the course of treatment can change, so can your doctors. You are in charge of your body. It is always your decision.

Many patients don't realize that they don't have to settle for the first doctor assigned to them.

Just as you might be given a certain medication, only to later learn you're allergic to it. In that instance, the course of treatment will change. You don't have to take any medication you don't feel comfortable taking. It's the same thing with choosing your healthcare providers. If the doctor or medical staff you've been assigned isn't the right fit for you, it is 100% your human right to ask for someone new. If I had stayed with my first doctor, I would be in the ground right now, instead of being here trying to help keep you out of the ground too. I owe my life to my medical team, specifically my Cardiologists, Dr. Alberta L. Warner, MD with the West Los Angeles VA Hospital, and Dr. Michelle M. Kittleson, MD at Cedars Sinai. Flat out, I would not be here today if not for them. They and their medical institutions, in my opinion, are true champions of pa-tience and understanding that we all come from different circumstances. The biggest difference between Dr. Warner and Dr. Kittleson, and my first doctor is they listened to me, worked with my care-takers, social workers, and we came up with my healthcare plan together. When the time came to execute that game plan, we were all on the same page and we won. I know we won, because I'm here working to get you to win one as well.

Secret #3:

Be prepared for a psychological examination and to lose weight.

It doesn't matter who your doctor is, trust me when I tell you, from the moment any doctor meets you they are evaluating you. Your mental health goes a long way in terms of determining your fate, especially if you are being considered for an organ transplant. How doctors perceive you on every visit is highly important. They are tracking all of your progress and if they have any mental health concerns, you can have your request for an organ transplant be denied.

Essentially a death sentence, but luckily for you, so long as you can show a willingness to follow instructions and work with your team, it doesn't have to be. A lot of people think they can advocate for themselves, but working with your team to educate yourself about what goes into a psyche exam can be your difference maker.

Another thing that patients need to know is that every person who receives a heart or kidney transplant will be required to lose weight. It's just one of many things that you will be required to do prior to any procedure. The doctors want to make sure you can follow instructions and aren't

wasting everybody's time, and more importantly, wasting an organ that could go to someone who will treat the process with the seriousness that it deserves. You need to want to make it as well. You need to want to be involved, engage your doctor, ask questions. If every time a doctor sees you, you're lying in the bed and not working at getting out of it or uninterested in going through the necessary steps to get better, all of that will be factored into the doctor's decisions being made about you. Trust the process, but involve yourself and your team in the process, every step of the way. Winners need to know what play to run in order to win. That's why everyone needs to communicate.

Secret #4:

Educate yourself about EKG's and what they entail before going into the hospital and stay relaxed.

The most important way for doctors to know what is going on with you is to have you go in for an EKG. Many people today don't know the condition of their heart and It's very important for them to know the shape of their heart and how it is working. An EKG is the best and safest method for achieving that, but the problem is that they are intimidating to the average person.

They're also very long and both physically and mentally taxing, but I think if EKG's were more openly discussed and patients were better prepared to experience them, they wouldn't be so resistant to having them done. The reality is, an EKG is the best thing for your heart's health.

They let the doctors know what's really going on with you and better inform them to manage your healthcare.

Everyone has their own preparation process, but in my case, it was important for me to be as relaxed as possible. I'm normally a very friendly and talkative person, but for me, prior to an EKG is not the time for small-talk. I needed to prepare myself to be quiet for a long time. Most doctors and nurses like to chat with you before going, but I had to let them know, "from this point on, can we please not talk, so I can stay relaxed and keep my heart rate as even as possible?" It's okay for you to do that too. If anything, they will appreciate the respect you have for the procedure.

Secret #5:

Blood and urine don't lie.

Just the same, as the results of an EKG, the best thing you can do for yourself when you go to the doctors is request that they test your blood and urine. A blood and urine test is even easier than an EKG. If you're feeling even the slightest bit off, request that the lab check your blood and urine. Nowadays if you know where the lab is and you are familiar with how everything works, they can test your blood and urine before you even see your doctor. The results can take time, so you have to be patient, but it undoubtedly allows you and your medical team to make informed decisions about managing your healthcare faster than they would if you weren't. When it comes to healthcare, timing is everything and anyway that you can save your healthcare providers time, only works out in your favor. Trust me.

Secret #6:

You're the quarterback, your Doctor is Your Coach, now create your dream team.

There is nothing more important in the relationship between a patient and their healthcare providers than trust. If you don't trust your doctors then you are just wasting your time. The first doctor I ever had, sent me home to die. Straight up. He didn't trust that I could live and I didn't trust his medical judgement. We weren't the right fit for each other, clearly. I should have trusted my gut instinct then, and asked for a new doctor, but I didn't know. I've had many doctors since then. Some great and some not so great. The important thing is where I am now with my medical team. I trust Dr. Kittleson at Cedars and Dr. Warner at the VA with my life. We have a mutual respect for one another and that is the only reason why my relationships with them have

been able to flourish. I worked with Dr. Warner for years to get my body ready to receive a transplant. It didn't happen overnight. We came up with a plan and I followed it. 6 months before I was approved, I was sent to Dr. Kittleson and we worked together to get us across the finish line. I say "us", because when I got my transplants, it wasn't just me, it was a win for our whole

team. I was the quarterback and they were my coaches. We won together.

In closing...

Upon reading this pamphlet, if you would like to read more, I have a book available, detailing my full experience and my journey from medical mistrust to patient advocacy. Beyond that, if you're ready, you can take the next steps in creating your dream team for managing your healthcare, by making a profile at our website **www.win-one.org/theemiracle-mann.** *By simply entering your address, you can be linked with doctors and social workers in your area that can get you the help you need now. You can also enter the contact information for all the members of your team, ensuring that there are no lapses in communication and everyone is on the same page.*

If you feel you need more support and would like to speak directly with people who have gone through or, are currently going through a similar health situation as you are now, please consider joining one of our regularly occurring online support groups, or come participate in one of our Win-One workshops. **"Thee Miracle Mann Program"** *is a resource for anyone who considers themselves not highly educated, and anyone who feels* *like they don't fully understand, "Doctor speak". It's for people who have gone through an unexpected or traumatic illness, for people who are clueless on who to trust and how to determine who to trust, and for the individuals who don't fully realize their rights as a patient, or have currently been assigned an old school doctor, but really need a doctor, who embraces new school thinking. Most folks don't realize that they need to be the ones managing their healthcare. They need to be their own quarterback and that's what this program is about. I want to empower you to be the quarterback of your team the same way I am of mine.*

The next step, once you have created your team, is following through on your game plan. I wish I had someone to teach me the way I am teaching you. This will cut years out of the process and in the long run get more people seeking organ transplants to be considered as legitimate prospects for the programs available at Cedars and the VA.

Follow the steps and we can win one together!

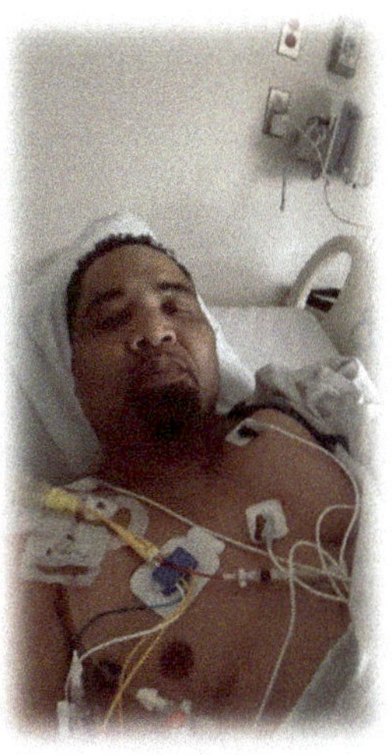

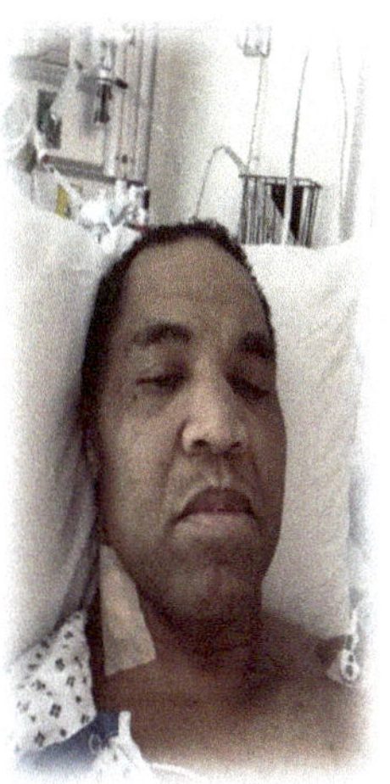

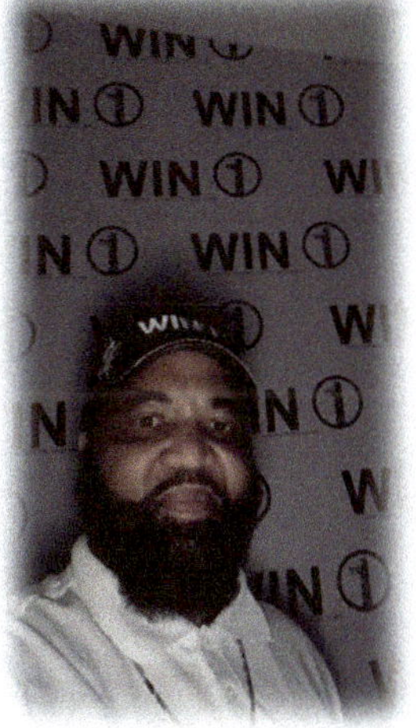

WIN 1
WIN 1   WIN 1
WIN 1   WIN
WIN 1   WIN
WIN   WIN 1
WIN 1
N 1   WIN 1
WIN 1

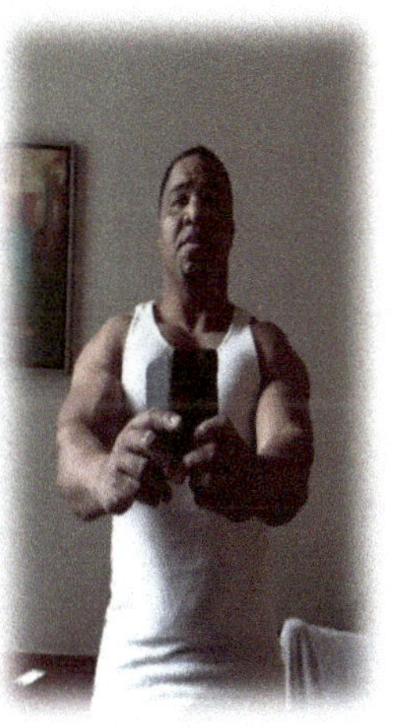

"CHOOSING THE RIGHT CAREGIVER IS NOT JUST A DECISION; IT'S AN ACT OF LOVE AND TRUST."

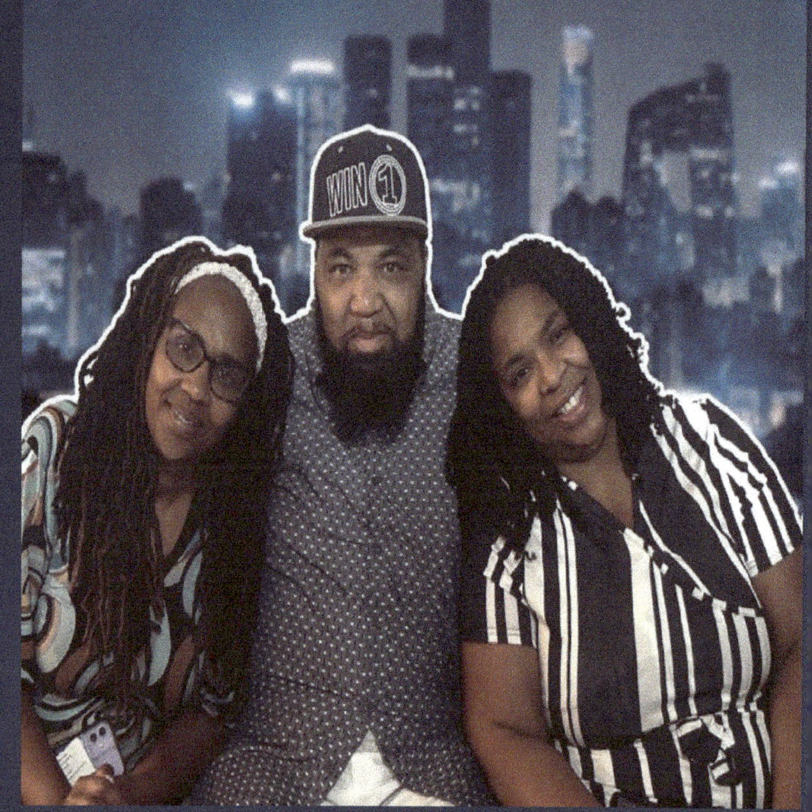

Caregiving Tasks

PATIENT

DATE

M T W T F S S

CARERS

CAREGIVER NAME	START TIME	END TIME

FOOD / DRINK

MEAL	DESCRIPTION	✓	TIME
BREAKFAST			
LUNCH			
DINNER			

SNACKS			LIQUIDS		

HYGIENE

TASK	✓
SHOWER / BATH	
BRUSH TEETH (MORNING)	
BRUSH TEETH	
CHANGE CLOTHING	

HOUSE HOLD TASKS / CLEANING

TASK	✓

HEALTH

TASK	✓
BLOOD SUGAR TEST	
BLOOD PRESSURE TEST	

EXERCISE / ACTIVITY

ACTIVITY	✓

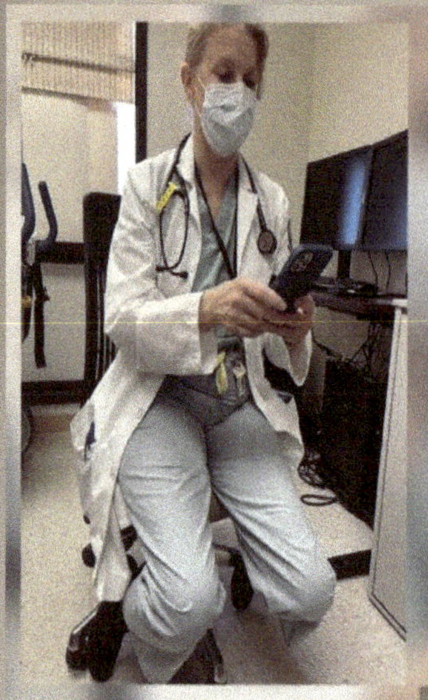

QUARTERBACK
ELITE COACH

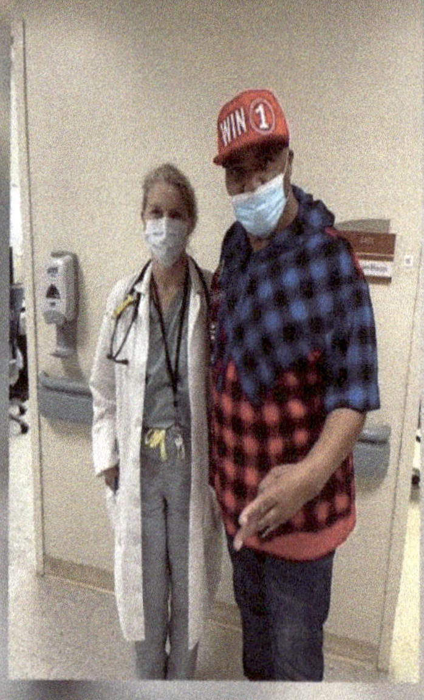

QUARTERBACK
ELITE COACH
WIN 1

Teach me how to Win in the Medical World.

After experiencing hospice twice, I resolved to return to the Los Angeles VA hospital and consult with Dr. Alberta Warner. Placing my complete trust in her, I found solace in her tears upon my arrival. Dr. Warner, a beautiful soul with both education and compassion, treated me not as a routine patient but as the chosen one for that moment. Together, we embarked on the journey of crafting a brand new day and formulating a successful plan for the future.

Allergy- Family DNA
A condition in which the immune system reacts abnormally to a foreign substance.

MOST COMMON TYPES
Drug allergy
An abnormal reaction of the immune
system to a medication.

Food allergies
An unpleasant or dangerous immune
system reaction after a certain food is
eaten.

Contact dermatitis
A skin rash caused by contact with a
certain substance.

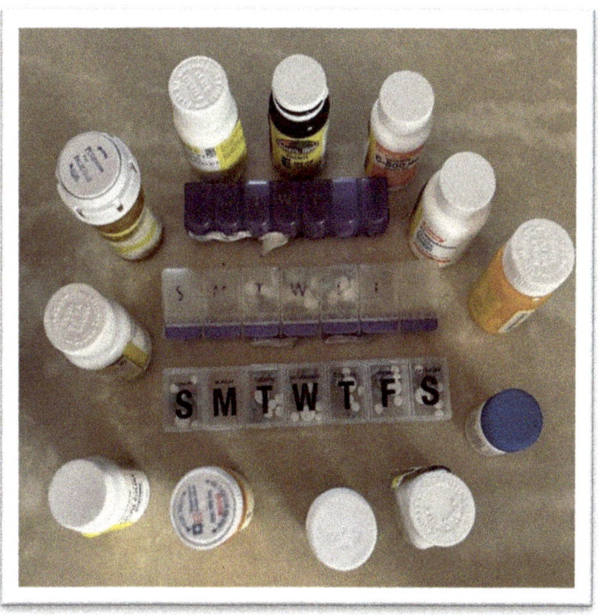

It's a valuable practice to inform your doctor that you manage your medication independently, including awareness of dosage times and potential side effects. dosage times and potential side effects.

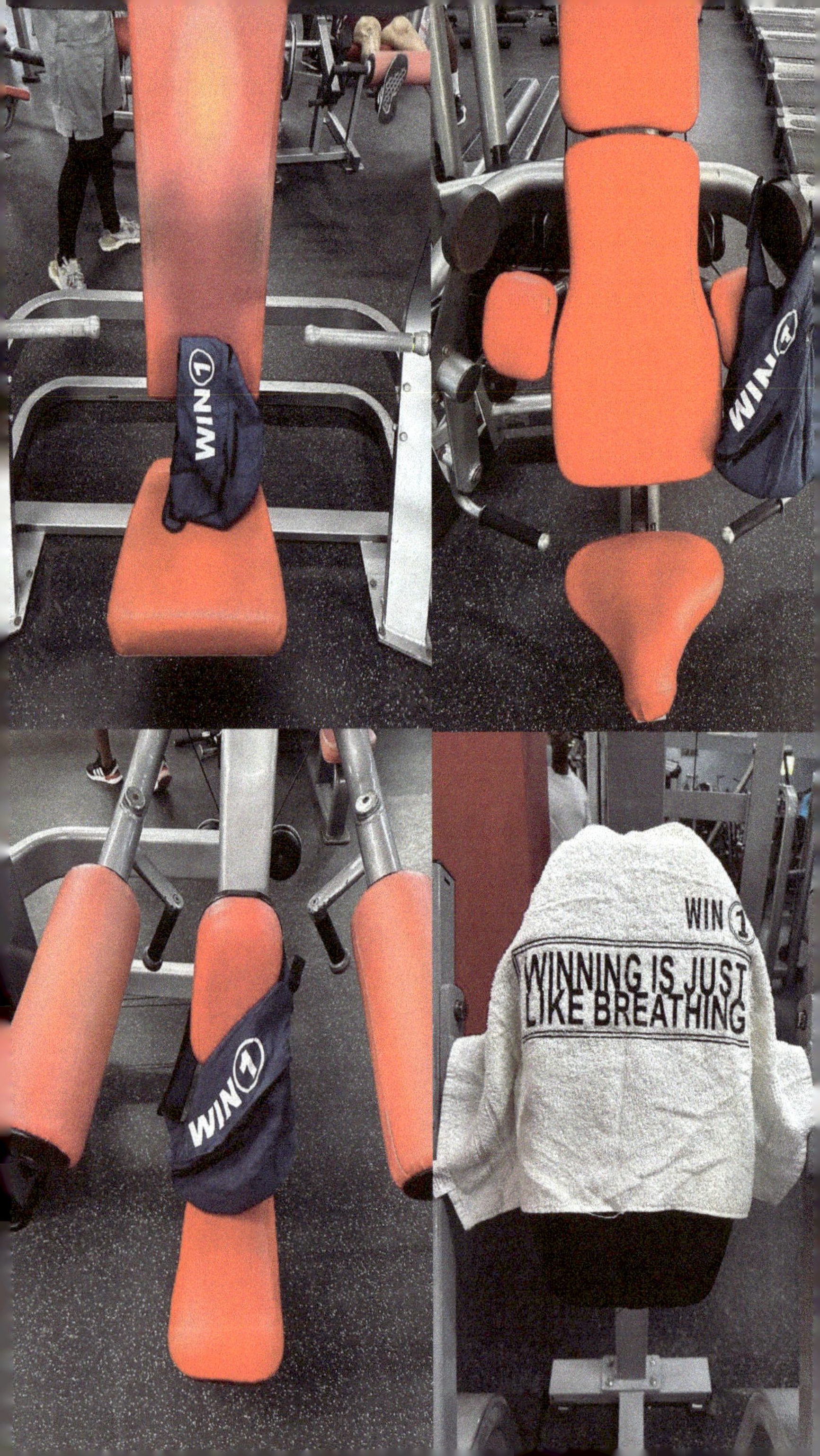

WIN 1
WIN 1
WIN 1
WIN 1
WINNING IS JUST LIKE BREATHING

Individuals can achieve a transformation in their body composition by engaging in a well-rounded fitness regimen. Combining cardiovascular exercises to burn fat with strength training to build muscle can lead to a leaner and more toned physique. As one loses fat through activities like aerobic exercise, and simultaneously engages in muscle-strengthening exercises, the overall appearance of the body may change, giving the impression of a conversion from fat to muscle. Nonetheless, it's essential to recognize that these processes occur independently, and the key lies in striking a balance between fat loss and muscle gain for a healthier and more fit body.

Make the MOVE! Weight Management Program, supported by VA's National Center for Health Promotion and Disease Prevention (NCP). We at NCP are proud to make this program available to our Veterans. Now in its second decade, MOVE! includes the most up-to-date approaches for weight management. Please explore our website to learn more about MOVE!

http://www.move.va.gov/

"Eating to live" encapsulates the philosophy that views food as essential fuel for sustaining life rather than a mere indulgence. This perspective emphasizes nourishing the body with a balanced and nutritious diet, prioritizing health and well-being. The focus shifts from consuming for pleasure or habit to making mindful choices that support overall physical and mental vitality. By recognizing the profound impact of nutrition on longevity and quality of life, individuals adopting an "eating to live" approach often make choices that prioritize nutrient-dense foods, promoting longevity and sustained well-being. In essence, this philosophy encourages a conscious and purposeful relationship with food, aligning dietary habits with the goal of fostering a healthy and resilient life.

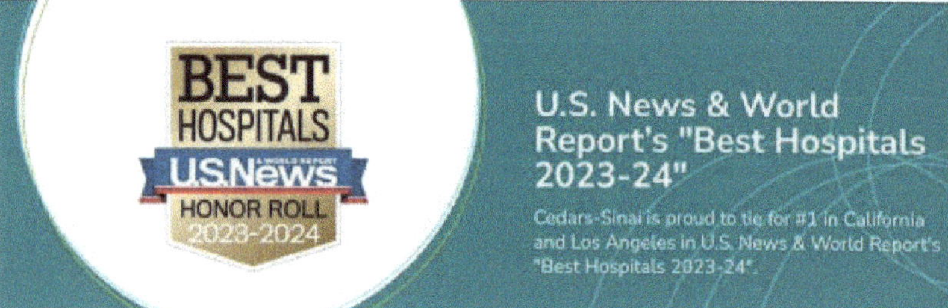

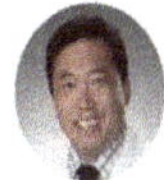

Richard T. Kim, M.D.

📞 (916) 325-1040

📍 1508 Alhambra Blvd.
Suite 200
Sacramento, CA 95816

Critical Care Medicine
✓ Accepting new patients

Pulmonary Disease
✓ Accepting new patients

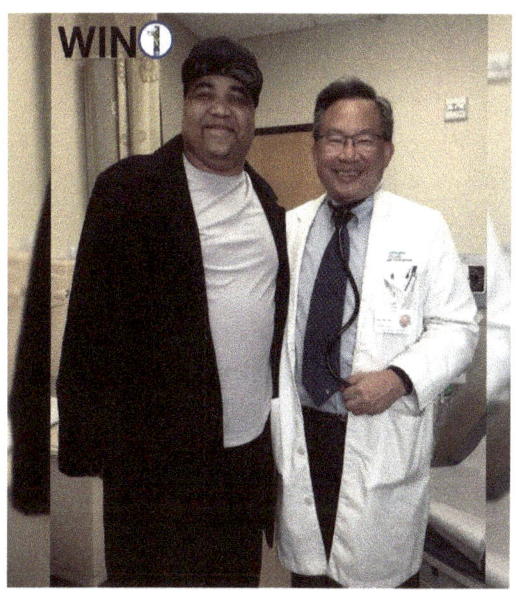

Opting for a new medical doctor can be a pivotal decision. It may arise from various reasons, such as seeking a fresh perspective on your health, desiring a different approach to treatment, or even relocating to a new area. This transition allows for a renewed focus on your well-being and ensures that your healthcare aligns with your evolving needs and preferences.

Mental Health

Receiving mental health support within the confines of an ICU room is a nuanced experience that highlights the interconnectedness of physical and mental well-being. In these critical settings, patients often grapple not only with the immediate challenges of their physical health but also with the emotional toll of the circumstances. Mental health professionals play a crucial role in providing support, offering a compassionate presence and tailored interventions to address the psychological impact of intensive care. Whether through counseling, mindfulness techniques, or collaborative discussions with the medical team, integrating mental health care into the ICU setting aims to holistically address the complex needs of patients, recognizing the profound link between emotional resilience and the healing process during times of medical crisis.

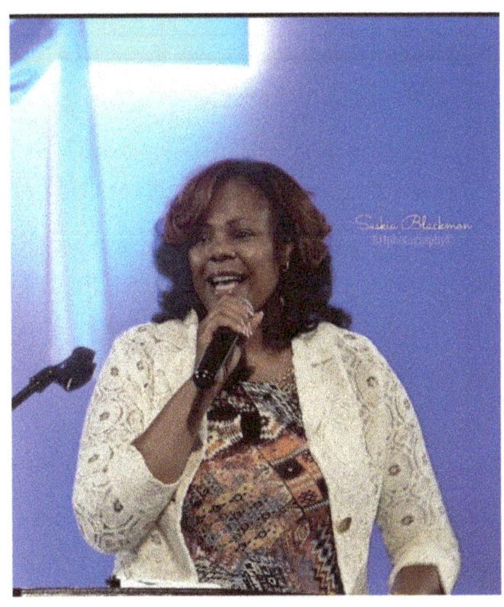

Lady'Dollye Stallworth-Dockery

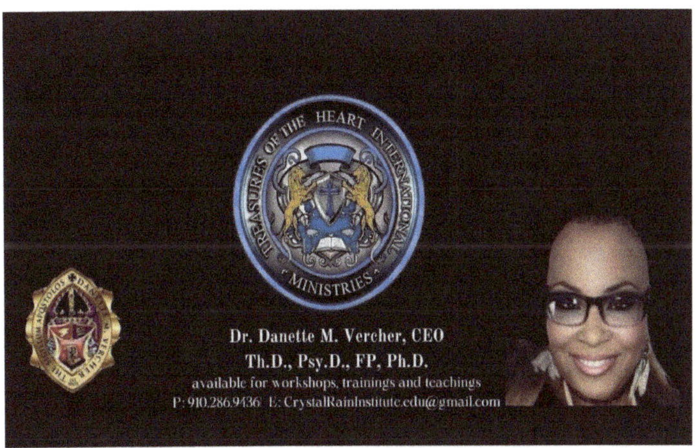

Dr. Danette M. Vercher, CEO

available for workshops, trainings and
teachings
P: 910.286.9436 E: CrystalRainInsti-
tute.edu@gmail.com

Privacy in the ICU room, for a patient, becomes a delicate yet essential aspect of their healthcare experience. The ICU is inherently an intense and vulnerable environment, where individuals often grapple with critical health conditions. Balancing the need for vigilant medical care with the patient's right to privacy is crucial. In this setting, respecting personal boundaries, confidential conversations, and maintaining dignity become integral components of quality healthcare. Patients deserve a sense of autonomy, even in their most challenging moments, and healthcare providers strive to create an atmosphere that safeguards their privacy, fostering trust and ensuring that the patient's dignity is upheld throughout their medical journey in the ICU.

Ensuring a consistently clean room in the ICU is paramount for both patient well-being and infection control. Daily maintenance involves rigorous sanitation protocols, prompt disposal of medical waste, and meticulous cleaning of surfaces. This commitment to cleanliness not only promotes a safe and hygienic environment for patients with compromised health but also minimizes the risk of hospital-acquired in fections. Healthcare professionals diligently adhere to stringent cleaning routines, emphasizing the importance of a pristine ICU setting to support the recovery and overall health of patients under their care.

Maintaining a positive attitude in the ICU is a formidable challenge met with unwavering determination by both patients and healthcare professionals. Amidst the clinical machinery and serious health conditions, optimism serves as a powerful catalyst for healing. Patients draw strength from the encouragement of dedicated healthcare providers, creating a supportive atmosphere that transcends the clinical setting. The resilience exhibited in fostering a positive mindset is not only a coping strategy but a beacon of hope, influencing the overall well-being of individuals navigating through critical health moments. It is a collective effort that transforms the ICU into a space where positivity becomes a vital component of the healing process, fostering a sense of strength and possibility amidst medical challenges.

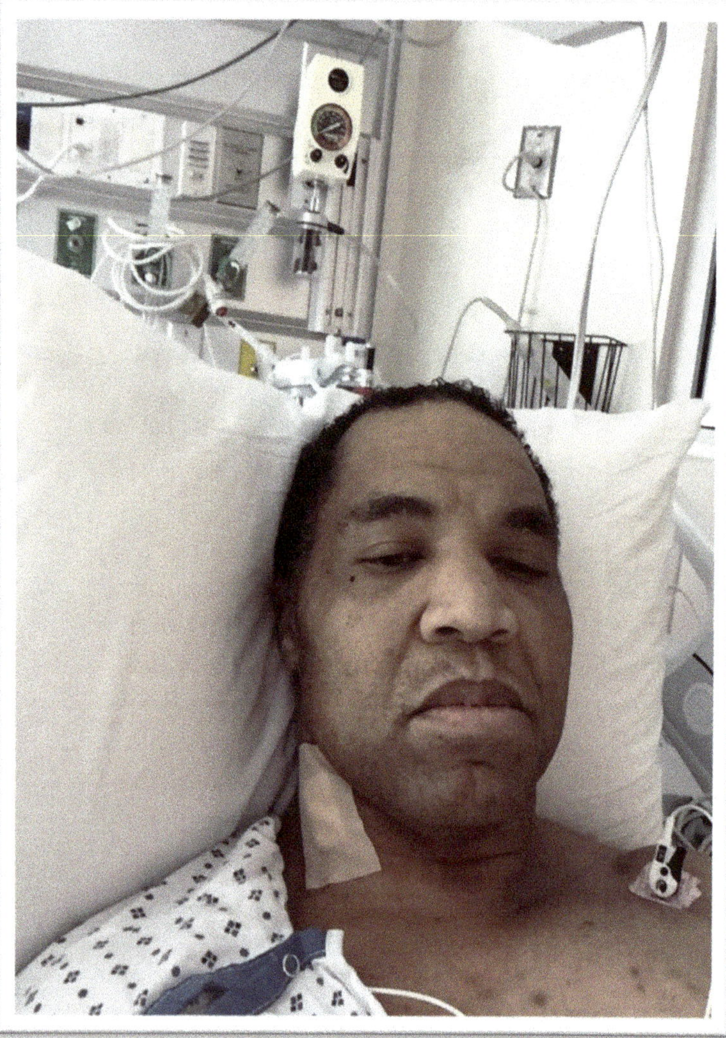

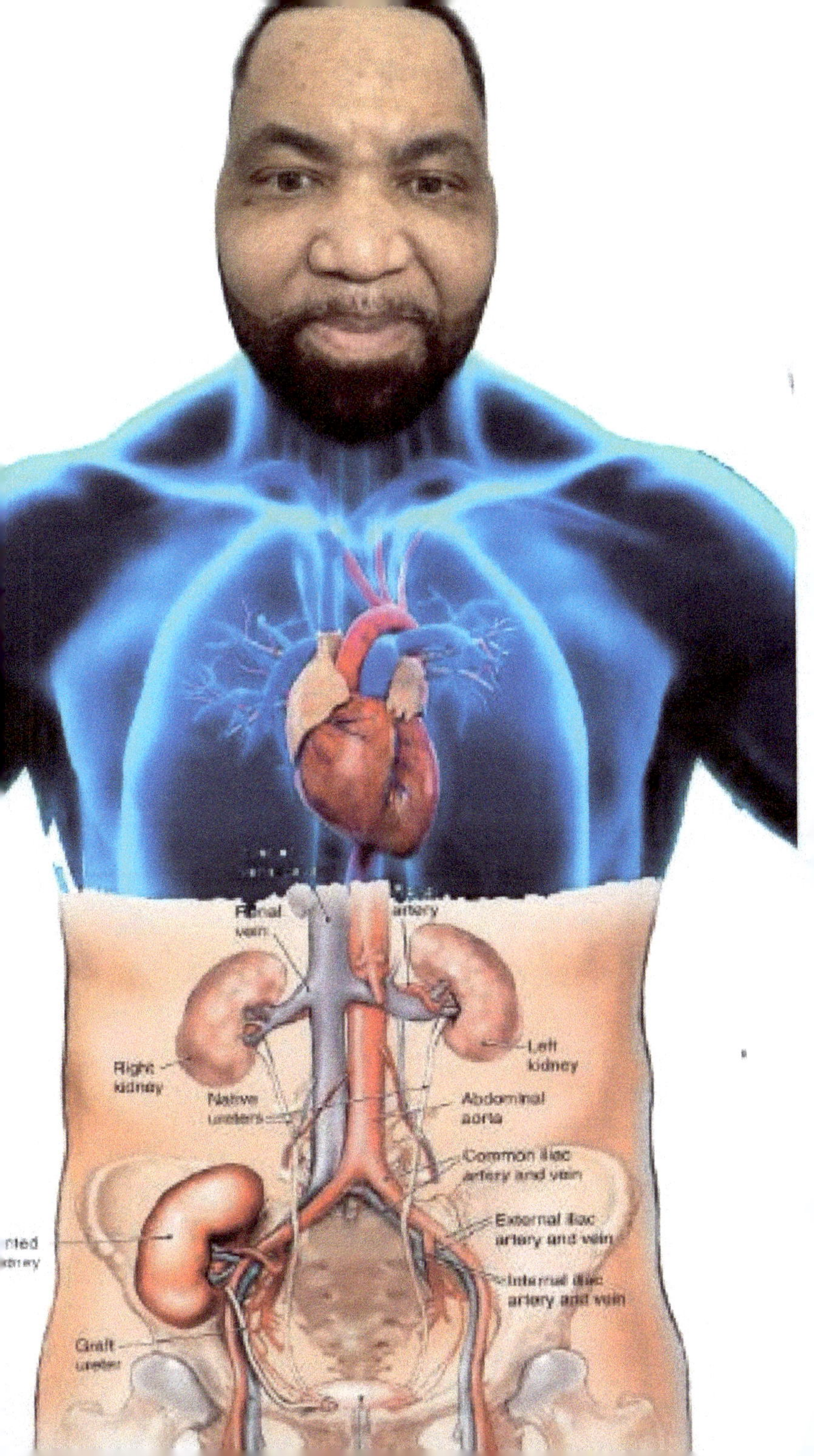

Renal vein
Renal artery
Right kidney
Native ureters
Left kidney
Abdominal aorta
Common iliac artery and vein
External iliac artery and vein
Internal iliac artery and vein
Graft ureter

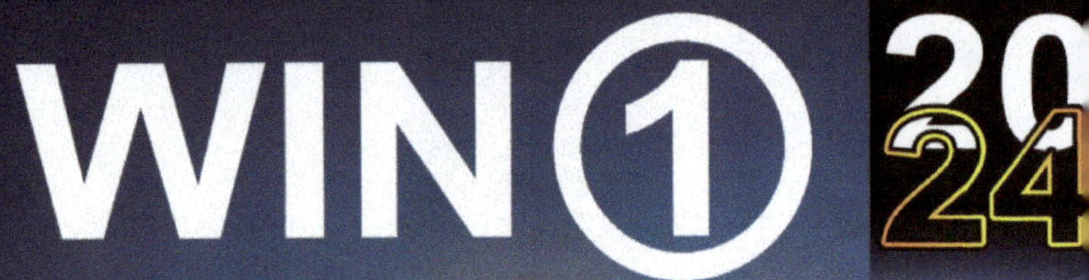

WIN ①
2024

JANUARY

Doctor's Notes

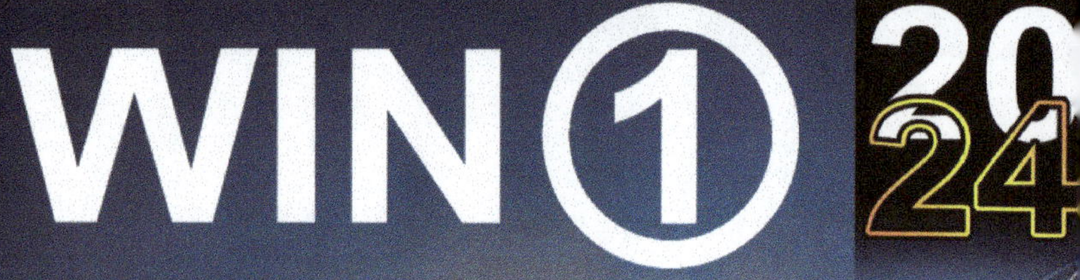

WIN ①
2024
FEBRUARY

Doctor's Notes

WIN ① 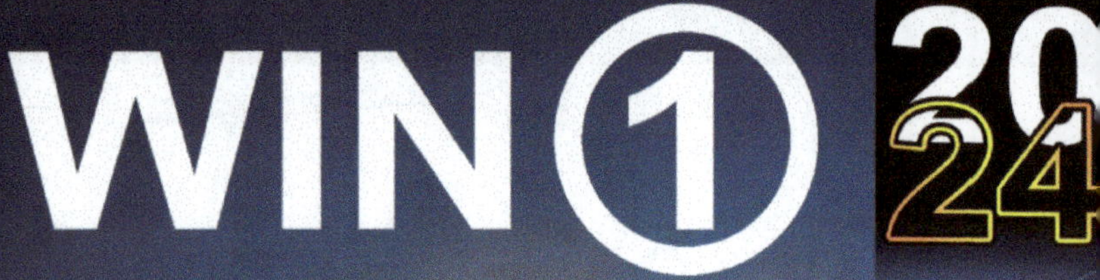

MARCH

____
____
____
____
____
____
____
____
____
____
____
____

Doctor's Notes

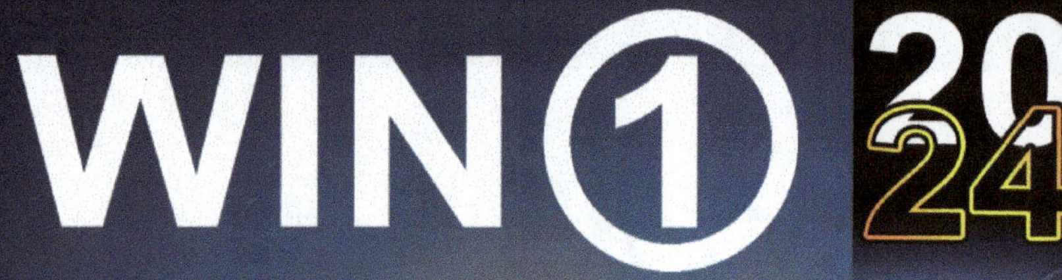

APRIL

Doctor's Notes

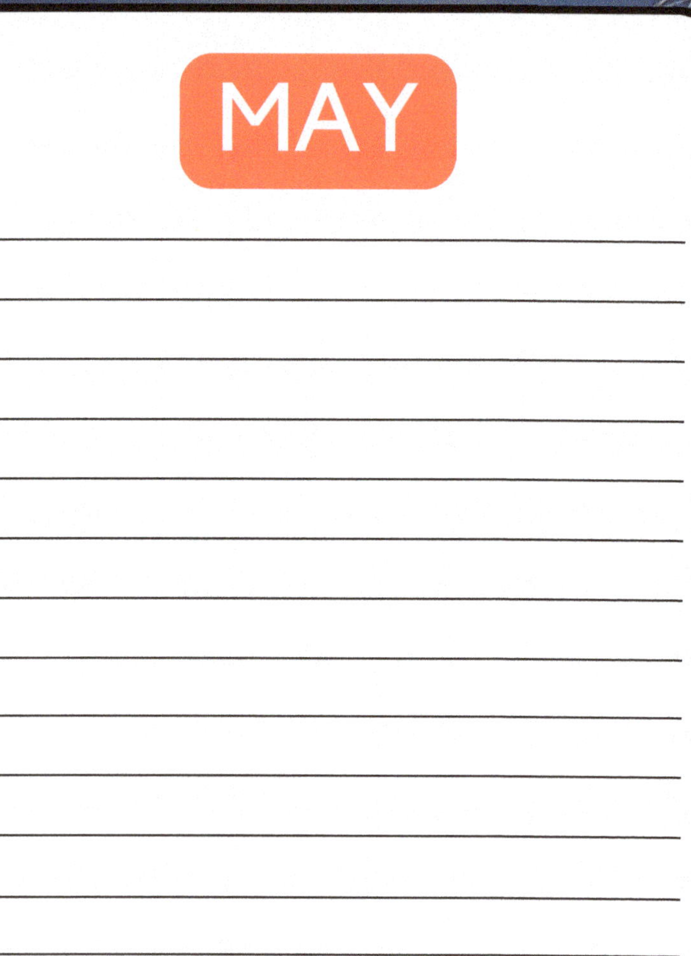

WIN 1
2024
MAY

Doctor's Notes

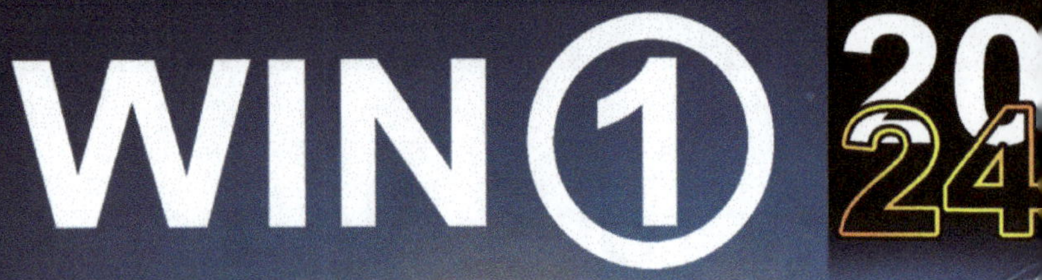

WIN ① 20 24

Doctor's Notes

WIN ① 2024

Doctor's Notes

WIN ①

AUGUST

Doctor's Notes

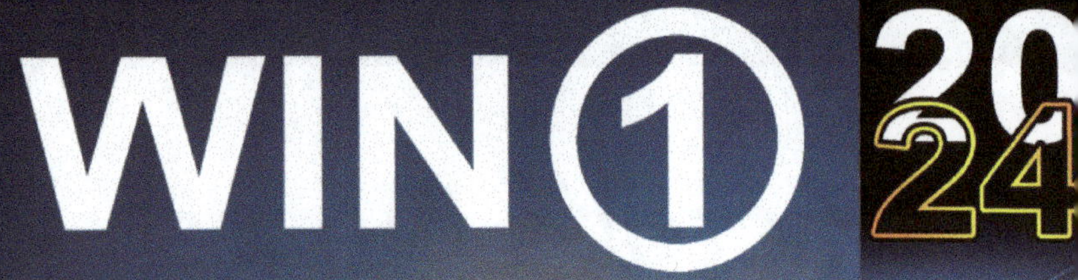

SEPTEMBER

Doctor's Notes

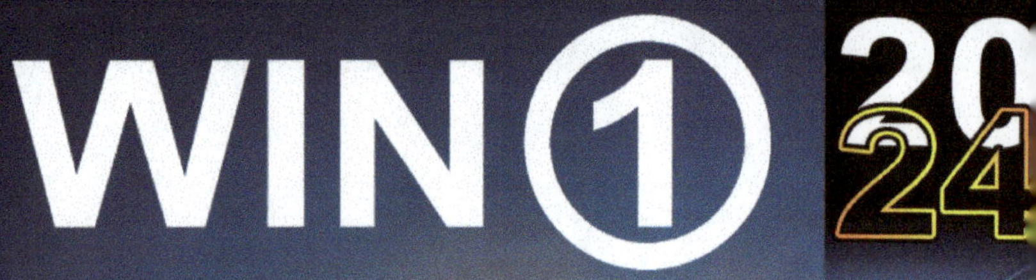

OCTOBER

Doctor's Notes

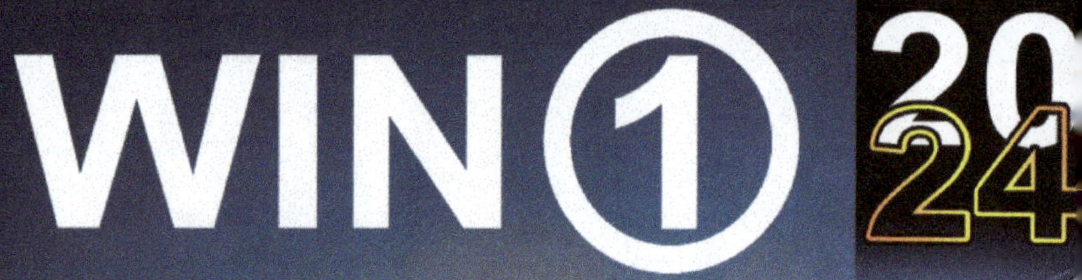

WIN 1
2024

NOVEMBER

Doctor's Notes

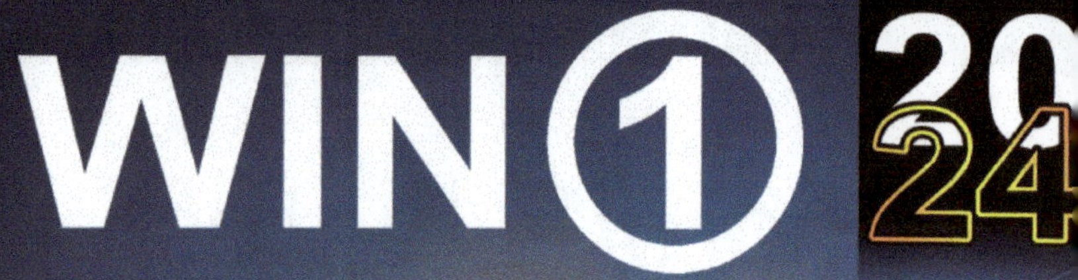

DECEMBER

Doctor's Notes

WIN 1

SIX SECRETS FOR SURVIV-ING THE ICU